Diabetes on Quest & Ans

(An awareness initiative for people in general)

by
Dr. Dulal Saha
Coochbehar, West Bengal, India

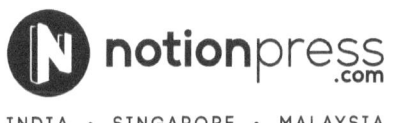

INDIA • SINGAPORE • MALAYSIA

Notion Press Media Pvt Ltd

No. 50, Chettiyar Agaram Main Road,
Vanagaram, Chennai, Tamil Nadu – 600 095

First Published by Notion Press 2021
Copyright © Dr. Dulal Saha 2021
All Rights Reserved.

ISBN 978-1-63850-878-6

This book has been published with all efforts taken to make the material error-free after the consent of the author. However, the author and the publisher do not assume and hereby disclaim any liability to any party for any loss, damage, or disruption caused by errors or omissions, whether such errors or omissions result from negligence, accident, or any other cause.

While every effort has been made to avoid any mistake or omission, this publication is being sold on the condition and understanding that neither the author nor the publishers or printers would be liable in any manner to any person by reason of any mistake or omission in this publication or for any action taken or omitted to be taken or advice rendered or accepted on the basis of this work. For any defect in printing or binding the publishers will be liable only to replace the defective copy by another copy of this work then available.

Presented to:

....
....
....

Dedication

It is said that God is omnipotent, omniscient and omnipresent but is unseen. We have observed in times few godly personalities used to come in the earth whom we call as prophet who are normally friend, philosopher and guide of everyone. I pay my whole hearted regard to each of them. Today, I am offering this little book at the lotus feet of my Lord, the Ideal, the most beloved – SriSri Thakur Anukul Chandra, the founder of Satsang, a socio-religious and cultural organisation who has demonstrated the principle of life throughout His life and left behind number of massages for 'being and becoming of life' for every one of us. Let He be pleased and make everyone be pleased.

Contents

Introduction   9
Acknowledgement   11

1. Diabetes & Introduction   13
2. Diabetes and Diet   17
3. Diabetes and Exercise Practices   26
4. Diabetes & Treatment   32
5. Pregnancy and Diabetes   36
6. Diabetes and Monitoring   46
7. Diabetes and Hypoglycaemia   52
8. Diabetes and Complication   58
9. Diabetes and Obesity   70
10. Diabetes and Special Situations   72
11. Diabetes and Future   76

Introduction

Diabetes is a chronic metabolic disorder and its increasing nature is mostly responsible for rapid urbanisation, irregular life style, diet habit and mental distress.

Now a days, I feel, Diabetes is known by all of us as because its prevalence is increasing rapidly. In urban area about 10 to 14% and in rural area about 3 to 7% are suffering from Diabetes and total population in India is about 73 million among 20 years and above with a much higher prevalence among individual aged over 50 years as per INDIAB study in last October 2019.

The diabetic not only gets sufferings but gets a reoccurring expenditure and if complication sets in then expenditure increases many folds. Along with sufferings and disability it produces a tremendous economic burden to the individual, family and as well as to the society. It is seen that medical expenditure for a Diabetic is about 2.5 folds higher than a non-Diabetic.

Hence, it requires a special attention and planning and awareness among all types of people. **Dr. P. Elliot Joslin**, the founder of Joslin clinic, Boston, US, commented- **"The diabetic who knows the most, lives the longest"** And **Prof. Dr. M. Viswanathan**, the founder of M.V. Hospital for Diabetes and Diabetes Research Centre, Chennai, India used to say- "**Early detection of Diabetes is the best form of Diabetes prevention and good control of Diabetes is the way to prevention of complication**". But it requires a tremendous effort, help and assistance among all classes of people.

The present book- **"Diabetes on Quest and Ans"** is a little forward in this regard. If it helps a little then the effort will be regarded as success.

Date: 1.3.2021   Dr. Dulal Saha

E mail: drdulalsaha@gmail.com

Acknowledgement

I must forward my heartful thanks to my patients and their attendant who have asked most of the questions in my clinic and to the people who has attended and asked question in various Diabetes awareness camp. I also, forward my special thanks to them who have encouraged me to publish in book form. It is needless to thank my family members who has help me a lot directly and indirectly for such involvement. My special thanks to the people of notion press and publishing house who has made the book in reality. I hope and pray for good for everybody.

Date: 1.3.2021　　　　　　　　　　　　Dr. Dulal Saha

Diabetes & Introduction

1. **Quest**: How one can understand that one has Diabetes? What are the primary symptoms?

   Ans: The initial symptoms of diabetes are excess thirst, frequent urination, excessive hunger. As a result, there is a loss of body weight, weakness, muscle cramp, burning sensation in the hands and feet, delayed wound healing etc.

2. **Quest**: Is diabetes curable?

   Ans: No, it is not curable but it can be kept under control and can live a normal life like other people.

3. **Quest**: How to control diabetes?

   Ans: When the primary symptoms of diabetes develop, one should not waste time to consult a doctor. In the initial stage, food planning and exercise is sufficient to control diabetes. Sometime medicine may require.

4. **Quest**: How long a patient should take medicine for diabetes? Is it life long?

   Ans: As it is not possible to cure diabetes completely, so one has to take medicine for lifelong. The main object is to keep blood sugar under control. So, one has to follow the diet plan, exercise and medicine as per advice of the doctor.

5. **Quest**: Why diabetes develops? Whether any particular organ is responsible?

   Ans The main responsible organ for diabetes is Pancreas. It remains behind the stomach in our belly. The pancreas contains a special type of cells named beta cells of Langerhans which produces Insulin. This insulin facilitates entry of sugar into the cell from blood and thus maintain a normal blood sugar level. Deficiency of insulin or absence of insulin causes diabetes or high blood sugar.

6. **Quest**: Whether Diabetes are of different types?

   Ans: Yes, diabetes mainly of two types. Type-1 and type-2. Almost 90% percent of the diabetics are of Type 2 variety. Usually it appears in older age, after the age of 30 to 35 years. It usually runs in family. Type 1 diabetes usually occurs in children. Their beta cells of pancreas are destroyed in some unknown causes. So, in this case, from the beginning of diabetes one has to take insulin. In addition, women during pregnancy sometime develops diabetes, they are termed as Gestational Diabetes. In some rare occasions, there is fibrosis or calcification usually following Chronic pancreatitis and they are termed as Fibro calculous pancreatic diabetes or FCPD.

7. **Quest**: What are the organs get damage from diabetes?

   Ans: Uncontrolled diabetes can harm every organs of the body. In Type-1 diabetes, complication usually appear after five years of detection. But in type 2 diabetes, complication starts even before the detection of diabetes.

8. **Quest**: Is diabetes hereditary?

   Ans: Yes, diabetes has hereditary influence, especially in the type-2 diabetes. However, environmental factors are equally important. The person of a diabetic family is like the gun loaded with bullet. It will not harm till the trigger is pulled. Pulling the trigger is the environmental effect. Environmental factors are any sort of extra pressure upon our body, for example, women during pregnancy, excess body weight (Obesity), wounds, heart-attack, some medicines, mental agony etc.

9. **Quest**: Is diabetes contagious?

   Ans: No, it is not contagious at all, even sharing food, free mixing or even with sexual contact.

10. **Quest t**: Is it possible to prevent diabetes?

    Ans: Total prevention of diabetes is possible – cannot be answered now. However, it is true that, the beginning of diabetes can be delayed. Those who are having family history of diabetes, if they follow the advises of a doctor, can postpone the occurrence of diabetes.

11. **Quest**: What other factors we need to control along with diabetes to prevent diabetic complication?

    Ans: High blood pressure, obesity, sedentary life style, high blood fats, tobacco use – all increase the diabetic complication in many folds. So, these things must also be controlled along with diabetes.

Diabetes and Diet

12. **Quest**: Whether diabetics can eat rice?

    Ans: Yes, surely, diabetics can take rice. 100gms of rice and 100gms of Atta, almost provides the same quantity of energy or calories. And they are bearing almost the same glycaemic index. So, rice or chapati (Roti) may be taken as one prefers – keeping mind on the quantity.

13. **Quest**: What is Glycaemic index?

    Ans: The carbohydrate containing food and glucose containing equal quantity of calories is given orally in two separate sittings and the blood is collected in half hour interval for two hours for blood sugar measurement. The difference or ratio between the two sets is the Glycaemic index of that food. Sugar or glucose is the smallest form of carbohydrate. So, the glucose absorption in the blood from the intestine is quick and easy. On the other hand, the more complex is the carbohydrate and more amount of diet fibre, the more delay is the rate of digestion and absorption. So, food having less glycaemic index is good for diabetes. Rice, wheat, barley etc. are of same glycaemic index.

14. **Quest** What is food fibre or dietary fibre?

    Ans: Dietary fibres are that component of food which is not digested, not produces calorie and have no nutritional value. It only increases the quantity of food. This is only present in vegetable food stuff. It prevents digestion of fatty meal, delays digestion and absorption of carbohydrates thus helps in diabetes and finally helps in formation in bulk or quantity of stool and help evacuation. Thus, those who are obese, has blood sugar, constipation etc., the dietary fiber acts as medicine.

15. **Quest**: What is calorie of food? What does it mean?

    Ans: Our body cell produces heat from the different components of food. The unit of that heat is called kilo calorie, in short, calorie. As for example, by breaking one gram of glucose produces four calories, from one gram of protein produces four calories and from one gram of fat produces nine calories.

16. **Quest**: What is the glycaemic index of potato? Can diabetics use Potatoes?

    Ans: Potatoes are full of carbohydrates and contains less amount of dietary fibre and gets digested easily. Thus, the glycaemic index is high and near to sugar or molasses and is about 80 to 90 percent. That is why restriction is given for potato. However, little quantity of potato along with other vegetables can be taken keeping eye on total quantity of calorie. The glycaemic index of potato and Taro is almost same. Sweet potato contains high amount of diet fibres and its glycaemic index is low, and is about 40 to 49 percent.

17. **Quest:** What about fruits? Do people with diabetes can take fruit?

    Ans: Keeping blood sugar under control, 100 to 150gms. of fruits of any variety can be taken. The fruits should be taken as a whole as much as possible. The fruits contain high number of fibres specially of soluble variety. It is found that blood sugar level gets peak sharper after taking juice of an apple then after taking whole apple.

18. **Quest**: Whether diabetics cannot take sugar at all?

    Ans: Sugar and glucose are the simplest form of carbohydrate. It requires no digestion. It gets absorbed instantly. Hence, it is restricted. However, according to the American diabetic Association, about 10 to 15 percent of total carbohydrate, one can take in the form of sugar. But it should be taken with other foods containing high dietary fibre.

19. **Quest**: Whether oil, ghee, butter has any restriction in diabetes?

   Ans: Butter and ghee are of animal origin and cooking oils are of vegetable origin. Animal fat contains cholesterol and saturated fat which are said to be harmful whereas vegetable oil contains unsaturated fatty acid which are not harmful rather protects from harmful effects of animal fat. High level of cholesterol and saturated fat deposits in the blood vessel causing obstruction in blood flow thus producing heart attack, stroke etc. Thus, who are having high cholesterol in blood, animal fat restriction is done for them. Otherwise, one teaspoonful of butter or ghee can be taken.

20. **Quest**: How is the amount of carbohydrate, protein and fat in the food should be?

   Ans: Food is measured in terms of calorie. Of the total calorie of food, the carbohydrate should contain about 50 to 60 percent, Protein should contain about 0.8 grams to 1.5 grams per kg of ideal body weight (according to the growth rate of the body) and Fat should contain about 20 to 30 percent, of which 2/3rd should come from vegetable fat and 1/3rd from animal fat. For example, if the total amount of calories of a person needs 2000, then, 60 per cent (2000 * 60/100 = 1200) i.e. 1200 calories should come from carbohydrate. As the calorie comes from 1 gm of carbohydrate is 4 calories, so the amount of carbohydrate is (1200/4 = 300) 300 grams. Again, rice and wheat contain 70% of carbohydrate, so to have 300gms of carbohydrate (100/70*300=430) 430 gm of rice or wheat can be consumed per day. In the same way fat will be (2000 * 30/100 = 600) 600 calories. And as 1 gm of fat produces 9 calories so fat requires (600/9 = 66), 66gms. And 1/3 of 66 grams that is 22gms should come from animal fat and 44gms should come from vegetable fat. The amount of protein in older cases, 0.8 grams per kg of ideal body weight and in the case of a child 1.5 grams per Kg of ideal body weight. The protein contains in the commonly used food items as cereals as rice / wheat (6 to 13%), pulses as dal (21 to 28%), Nuts (4.5 to 20%), Soya bean (43%), Fish (15–23%), Meat (18–26%), Egg (13%), Milk (3.2–4.3%) and vegetable and fruits (1–4%). As we are consuming 400gms of cereals so (8/100*400=32) 32gms of protein coming from that source. If we take at least 50gms of Dal (20/100*50=10) then another 10gms of protein is added. If we take milk or milk product of 250 ml of milk (4/100*250=10) then another 10gms of protein is added. Vitamin, minerals are plenty available in fruits and green leafy vegetables.

21. **Quest**: What is ideal body weight?

    Ans: If the height is measured in centimetre, then the ideal body weight will be, in case of male – (height in cm – 100) and in case of female, (height in cm − 100) * 0.9. If the height is measured in feet, the ideal body weight will be, in case of Male, for every 60 inches (5ft) 50 kg + for every inch 2.3 kg above 60 inches and in case of female for every 60 inches 45.5 kg + for every inch 2.3 kg above 60 inches.

22. **Quest**: Whether the diabetics can take Artificial sweetener such as Saccharin, Aspartame, Sucralose etc.? Are they harmful?

    Ans: Artificial sweetener as saccharin, aspartame, sucralose may be taken. No harmful affect is seen in human being in limited use.

23. **Quest**: Is there any diet list for a diabetic?

    Ans: Diet list is different for every diabetic. And the difference depends on age, height, nature of labour and life style. After calculating the total calorie of a person, most of the part is distributed in three main parts as breakfast, lunch and dinner and rest of the amount is distributed in between major meals as snacks. The diabetic should not take heavy meals at a time, frequent meal in every 3 to 3 +1/2 hours is good. The diabetic should not remain in empty stomach for long time as it may cause low blood sugar.

24. **Quest**: What about the underground vegetables as potato, carrot, radish, ginger, garlic, onion etc.

    Ans: Regarding the Potato and sweet potato is discussed in question no.16. Radish and carrot also can be taken in restricted amount. Ginger, onion and garlic, we use as spices in small amount, so there should not be restriction from diabetes point of view.

25. **Quest**: Can Diabetics take coconut and coconut oil.

    Ans: Coconut is a food of high food value. It contains high amount of oil and thus high calorie. The fat also contains saturated fat. So high intake may cause harm in cardio vascular system. So, in a restricted way we can consume coconut. Peanut also contains high amount of fat but not contains saturated fat.

26. **Quest**: Is there anymore restriction of diet for diabetics?

    Ans: From above discussion it is clear that there is no such restriction of food in diabetes. But it has some sort of plan. If the nondiabetics also follow the plan, they also can live healthy. If there is high blood pressure along with diabetes, then salt is made restricted. If there is damage in the kidney (renal insufficiency and renal failure) then, salt of sodium and potassium that is common salt and fruits and vegetables is made restriction. Apart from these conditions, there is no restriction of diet. If the nondiabetics also do suffer from such conditions, same types of restrictions are made for them.

27. **Quest**: Will You mention some food which a diabetic can take in plenty without any worry?

    Ans: Green leafy vegetables, green salad containing cucumber, tomato, carrot, lemon, green chilly etc, sprouted seeds are very good. Limited use of fruits is also good. They contain lot of vitamins, minerals, dietary fibres and antioxidants. Not only for diabetic persons, every person should consume those food regularly.

28. **Quest**: What is food pyramid?

    Ans: It is the graphic representation of food for Diabetes. Types of food which can be taken in plenty and what can be taken moderately or occasionally is arranged in pyramid shape. The food arranged in the bottom part of the pyramid can be taken in plenty and the food arranged on the top part can be taken in little amount and occasionally.

29. **Quest**: What is Diabetic food plate?

    Ans: In one 9inch dish the portion of carbohydrate, protein, vegetable is being distributed. In one diabetic dish almost 50% of dish should contain vegetables, green leafy vegetables and salad, 25% area should cover by carbohydrate containing food as rice, chapati, brown bread, dalia etc. and rest 25% of area should be occupied by protein and fat containing diet as dal, nuts, soya bean, fish, lean meat, egg and milk etc.

30. **Quest**: What is quantity of food per serving?

    Ans: The food grains as raw rice, dal, wheat etc. one serving= 30gms; in case of milk and fruit juice one serving = 120ml; in case of green vegetables, one serving = 2cups = 60gms; in case of ice cream, one serving = 2 t.s.f = 75gms

31. **Quest**: What is food substitute?

    Ans: It is the alternative choice of food keeping equivalent quantity and quality of food in terms of calorie, food fibers etc. For example, to choose chapati for rice.

Diabetes and Exercise Practices

32. **Quest**: Does practice of exercise essential in diabetes?

    Ans: Yes, exercise is one of the major components in the management of Diabetes. It is very difficult to control diabetes without exercise or sufficient labour.

33. **Quest**: How do exercise work?

    Ans: There are so many positive effects of exercise. They are as follows: 1. Reduction in body weight-There is contraction and relaxation of muscle in exercise and for these require energy which comes from breaking down of stored food (fat and glycogen) in muscle and fatty tissue and thus causing reduction in body weight. Along with exercise if there is dietary restriction then it becomes more affective. 2. Enhance action of Insulin – there are numbers of insulin receptors remain in the wall of every cell of our body which catches insulin and after several reactions sugar from blood enter into the cell. Those who are fatty and idle in nature, a portion of the insulin receptors remain inactive which on exercising become active and reduces the blood sugar level. 3. Reduces Total body fat – Regular exercise and control of diet reduces body fat and thus the bad fat for cardio vascular system as cholesterol, LDL and Triglyceride decreases where as good fat as HDL increases 4. Increases the capacity of heart and improves total circulatory system. 5. Controls Blood pressure. 6. Increases body's immunity. 7. Prevents cancer cell formation 8. Feeling of overall wellbeing in body and mind.

34. **Quest**: What type of exercises usually do good for diabetes?

    Ans: The aim of exercise is physical labour. And it should be in open air. The exercises where there is contraction and relaxation of muscles happen again and again as walking, running, jogging, swimming, skipping, free hand exercise, cycling – are all good for Diabetes.

35. **Quest**: Is it necessary to do exercise daily? How much it should be done?

    Ans: We can do exercise daily. If not possible, five days a week is must. 2 km walking or five km cycling in half an hour is sufficient. Running, jogging, skipping, swimming etc. for thirty minutes also can be done.

36. **Quest**: Whether, everyone can do any form of exercise?

   Ans: No, like medicine, type and duration of exercise also varies and is individualised. Depending on weight, age, diet and nature of job – exercise is suggested. Apart from these, the state of health and diseases of vital organs as eye, heart, liver, kidney and feet are also kept under consideration for exercise.

37. **Quest**: Sometimes, it is heard that strokes and heart attack happen while on exercise.

   Ans: It may happen. Hence it is advised that those who are specially above 30–35 yrs, before starting exercise they should first get check-up done by a doctor and as per advices of doctor they should start exercise. Initially one should start from light exercise as slow walking for 5 to 10 min and gradually to increase the limit and thus accident can be avoided.

38. **Quest**: Whether in pregnancy exercise can be done?

   Ans: Those who are habituated to perform exercise they can continue. New patients are not advised for exercise. But usual domestic work they can perform, if there is no restriction from Gynae doctor.

39. **Quest**: Sometimes patient cannot walk for diseases of back, leg or feet. In such case how patient will perform exercise?

Ans: In cases of diseases of limb, exercise should be done in such a way, so that, weight of body should not pass-through lower limbs. Cycling, swimming is good. And exercises which can be done in lying and sitting position are suitable for them. All the joints can be exercised avoiding the affected part or the part which causes pain. Of course, Doctor will guide.

40. **Quest**: Is there any bad effect of exercise?

    Ans: Irregular practice of exercise may cause harm. If exercise is done as per advices of a doctor, there should not be chance of having so. In general, it can be said that if there is any disease of vital organ as Liver, Kidney, Heart, Eyes etc doing hard exercise is not good. It is better to have suggestion from doctor before starting exercise.

41. **Quest**: Do you like to say anything more on exercise?

    Ans: Yes, there are so many points to note. Among them main points are: a) Those who are having very high blood sugar level and ill, they should first reduce their blood sugar level by taking medicine. b) Those who are taking medicine for diabetes, they should first take some light food as biscuits or puffed rice and water, otherwise there is a chance to develop low sugar symptoms. Hence, sometimes it is seen that on the way of performing exercise there is a sense of excess hunger, having excess sweating, feeling less energy to walk, even sometime gets senselessness. Hence, it is advised to take some snacks before starting exercise and carry some food as sugar candy, biscuits etc along with to avoid such dangerous events. c) When there is a situation to perform exercise or labour or hard work for long time as playing, they should eat some carbohydrate containing food in between. d) Patient should wear soft shoes as canvas or sports shoe to avoid foot injury.

42. **Quest:** Whether Yoga exercise has any good effect on Diabetes?

    Ans: Yoga-exercise has been practised in India as well as other parts of the world. From many observations, the effect of controlling blood sugar, blood pressure, blood fat, body weight and producing good sleep have been observed. After taking rest following some sort of free hand exercise, yoga practice provides best result. Tri konasana, Koti chakrasana, ardho bakrasana, Pawan muktasana, Surjya namaskar, Bhujangasana, dhonurasana, Pada chakrasana, shawasana are said to be very effective. Apart from these, the positive affect of Meditation, Prayer and Pranayam is also being observed. Those who have influence of diabetes in the family, if they practice physical exercise and Yogasana, then the onset of diabetes can be postponed. It is also observed that the dose of anti-diabetic medicines requires in less amount those who are doing regular exercise and Yogasana. They have a very good medicinal effect having no side effect or extra expenditure. Of course, it should be learned from a Yoga-master to get good result.

Diabetes & Treatment

43. **Quest**: The children with diabetes have to take insulin lifelong. Any other oral medicine can be replaced for insulin?

    Ans: No, Insulin is the best and only treatment in patient with Type 1 diabetes. No other medicine of any pathy is useful in controlling Diabetes.

44. **Quest:** Why it is so? Will you explain?

    Ans: In childhood diabetes, that is in Type 1 diabetes, the beta cells of pancreas from which insulin is secreted, are destroyed by some process leading almost total deficiency of insulin and thus causing high blood sugar. Hence Insulin from out-source is absolutely necessary. The other oral medicine usually works either through beta cell of pancreas or by activating the secreted insulin. As the beta cell is destroyed in type 1 diabetes where oral diabetic agent will act? And in practice also no result is experienced. Till date other option is to transplant beta cell of pancreas but not available yet.

45. **Quest**: Sometime, in older patient with Type 2 diabetes also used to take insulin.

    Ans: In type 2 diabetes Insulin is not always lifesaving but to maintain health and in special occasion insulin becomes necessary. The conditions where insulin becomes necessary are:

    1. when oral medicines in optimal dose cannot control blood sugar,
    2. Women in pregnancy state
    3. Before operation
    4. when there is disease involving the vital organs as Liver, Kidney, Lungs, heart, brain and nerves etc.
    5. complications out of diabetes. It is also observed that treatment with insulin is best and prevents complication best.

46. **Quest**: Whether medicines of Homeopathy and Ayurvedic can do good for Type 2 Diabetes?

    Ans: Yes, possible. But the affect and side-effect of the medicine should be scientifically proved. Because the aim of treatment of diabetes is not only bringing down the blood sugar but also to keep the patient healthy for now and future also.

47. **Quest**: Whether there is any side effect of orally taking anti diabetic medicine?

    Ans: The approved medicine itself has no such side effect causing disease of the vital organ. But if there is disease in vital organs then restriction is done in using oral anti diabetic medicine. Insulin is best in such cases.

48. **Quest**: Any side effect of Insulin?

    Ans: Presently available insulin as Human and analogue variety has no such side effect. But the rate of producing low sugar symptoms is more with insulin. It is the only side effect. Dose of insulin, diet plan and exercise or manual labour adjustment is required to overcome the problem.

49. **Quest**: As orally taking medicine, whether it may happen that with insulin also the blood sugar cannot be controlled.

    Ans: Usually blood sugar can be controlled with insulin. The dose of insulin depends on the production of insulin from the beta cell of pancreas. Less the production more insulin is required from out-source. But there is a condition called Insulin resistance where large quantity of insulin becomes necessary.

50. **Quest**: What is insulin resistance? Why it happens?

    Ans: When there is enough insulin in the body, even more than normal quantity and there is high level of blood sugar, in such condition it is called Insulin resistance. It is due to 1) Influence of some hormones as corticosteroid, Growth hormone, Oestrogen, Progesterone which prevents the action of Insulin 2) When a sufficient quantity of insulin receptors remains inactive.

51. **Quest**: Is it possible to overcome Insulin resistance?

    Ans: First we are to observe why it happens and then to manage the cause. In this way, in many instances it can be overcome.

52. **Quest**: Is it not possible to make oral preparation of Insulin?

    Ans: When we take insulin orally it is destroyed by acid of stomach. But scientists are trying – whether insulin can be taken in other routes. Now, Insulin nasal spray has come out but not yet available for use in general.

53. **Quest**: Is it must to keep insulin in fridge? Fridge is not available in many of our houses.

    Ans: If fridge is available, it is better to keep in fridge in the outer chamber not in deep fridge. Before using insulin, it is to be kept out for 10 to 15 minutes to bring down to room temperature. Insulin should not be given very cool. Those who have no fridge, they can keep the used insulin vial in cold and shaded place. Insulin should not be kept over hot articles and/or where sun shine falls. During travel it is better to carry in ice bag or in hand bag. In suitcase, it becomes hot.

Pregnancy and Diabetes

54. **Quest**: Is there any restriction to become mother in diabetes?

    Ans: No, no such restriction is there. Every woman can be a mother. Only thing is that blood sugar is to be controlled with insulin before conception and during pregnancy.

55. **Quest**: Most of the time, it is seen that there is miscarriage during pregnancy, sometime there is a birth of big baby and sometime with some sort of malformation in baby.

    Ans: Yes, it happens. Hence it requires a good control of blood sugar with 'Human Insulin'. Now a days 'Insulin Analog' is also successfully in use.

56. **Quest**: In Pregnancy, from when Insulin to be used?

    Ans: In diabetic women, the pregnancy or getting conception should be carried out in a plan. First, they are to consult with a physician experienced in diabetes and control of blood sugar is to be done by Insulin and other life style adjustment. After getting a green signal from Doctor, they will devote for conception. And Insulin to be continued to control blood sugar till the termination of pregnancy. Congenital malformations usually take place during 5 to 7 weeks of pregnancy. Hence, at that time the blood sugar is need to be controlled. If blood sugar remains high during pregnancy, then high amount of sugar gets entry in the foetus and deposited in the body and becomes big baby.

57. **Quest**: Why oral antidiabetic medicines are not in use in pregnancy?

    Ans: The oral antidiabetic medicine may lower the blood sugar of mother but when it enters into the foetal body, it also reduces the blood sugar of foetus. But Insulin is not getting entry into the foetal circulation from mother.

58. **Quest**: Why Human Insulin is asked to use?

    Ans: The structure of Human Insulin though made artificially are similar to Human's own Insulin. Other Insulin as Porcine and Bovine which are extracted from Pig and Bull, their structure is different from human insulin and thus when they are in use, they form a insulin anti body. This insulin antibody can easily enter into the foetal circulation and along with antibody, insulin also gets entry into the foetal circulation and causes lowering of foetal blood sugar. Now a days, porcine and bovine varieties of insulin are not in use. But a special designer insulin has come out and successfully are in use.

59. **Quest**: In women, sometime it is found that diabetes develops during pregnancy but disappears after pregnancy.

    Ans: When Diabetes develops during pregnancy it is called Gestational Diabetes (GDM). In such condition usually remains the influence of hereditary. During pregnancy there are different type of changes specially some hormonal changes which act against Insulin and Diabetes develop. But after delivery, the hormone level again sets to normal and Diabetes disappears.

60. **Quest**: Is treatment of GDM is similar to other type of pregnancy in diabetes?

    Ans: Yes, no oral diabetic medicines are usually given. If blood sugar is little bit high then diet plan and limited exercise is advised. When it is not controlled by diet and exercise, then human insulin is prescribed. If blood sugar is high in initial visits, then insulin is prescribed start with.

61. **Quest**: If quantity of food is made very less, whether there will be malnutritional effect on mother and baby.

    Ans: Diet plan or diet control does not mean less food. The quantity of food what require for a non-diabetic lady is also required for a diabetic lady. In addition, 300 calories extra require for the baby. Diet plan means when and what amount and type of food is necessary to maintain blood sugar without producing hypoglycaemia and to maintain overall nutrition for mother and baby.

62. **Quest**: What amount of exercise a pregnant diabetic lady should do?

    Ans: Those who are habitually performing exercise they can do. It is better not to start exercise in this stage. Normal work one can do. Walking for 20 to 30 minutes every one can do if there is no restriction from obstetrician.

63. **Quest**: What is the schedule of diabetes check-up in pregnancy?

    Ans: The pregnant women who have strong probability to develop diabetes but not developed symptoms of diabetes should get check-up for diabetes in first three months of pregnancy. If not detected at this time, then test to be repeated on 6th to 7th month. During pregnancy, if symptoms of diabetes as excess thirst, excess hunger, frequent urination or itching on genital part, she must inform Doctor and test for diabetes is to be done. Apart from this when goes for routine check-up for pregnancy, test for diabetes is also done.

64. **Quest**: Who are the persons who has strong probability to develop diabetes?

Ans: The high-risk persons to develop diabetes are: a. If there was diabetes in previous pregnancy. b. If there is family history of diabetes. c. If there is obesity or high body weight. d. If there is more increase in body weight in pregnancy e. If there is history of big baby in previous pregnancy. f. If there is history of early delivery in previous pregnancy. If any such above mentioned condition is there, blood sugar is done in first three months of pregnancy.

65. **Quest**: Is there any particular schedule to test for diabetes in pregnancy?

Ans: Blood sugar test is done as routine for every pregnant lady. If they have high risk of developing diabetes as discussed in previous question, their blood sugar is done even in first visit. They are given at random 50gms of glucose and blood sample is taken after one hour. If the blood sugar value becomes more than 140 mg/dl then three hours glucose tolerance test is advised. In such case, after collecting blood in fasting state in the morning, 100gms of glucose is given with a glass of water and after that every hour for three hours blood sample is collected. If the blood sugar value in fasting is 105 and after 1st, 2nd and 3rd hours value becomes 190 mg/dl, 165 mg/dl and 145 mg/dl respectively or more in any two values then the Gestational diabetes is said to be present.

66. **Quest**: What is the normal range of blood sugar in diabetes? Is it different from non-pregnancy state?

    Ans: Yes, it differs. In pregnancy state – Fasting-60 to 95 mg/dl, before meal (before lunch and dinner) 60 to 105 mg/dl and two hours after meal-120 mg/dl or less than 120 mg/dl and from 2 AM to 6 AM blood sugar should be kept above 60 mg/dl. If blood sugar falls down below 60 mg/dl, then body fat break down to form sugar and at that time ketone body is formed which is bad for baby's brain development. To avoid this situation, a bedtime snacks as a glass of milk and so, is essential.

67. **Quest**: How we can understand about the normal development of baby in the womb.

    Ans: First, we are to see about the status of blood sugar control. And it is done by

    1. frequent blood sugar check-up,

    2. Checking Fructosamine level which indicates average control of blood sugar in previous 7 days and

    3. Estimation of Glycosylated haemoglobin which indicates average blood sugar of previous 3 months. Secondly by observing the weight gain of mother. In first 3 months

there is increase in body weight from 1 kg to 2 kg, then in every week, there is increment of body weight by 350 to 400 gm and total gain in body weight about 10 to 12 kg till delivery. Apart from these, by doing Ultrasonography we can understand about the development of the baby in the womb.

68. **Quest**: Whether Caesarean section is must for pregnant lady? Normal delivery is not possible?

    Ans: If blood sugar remains under control, then usually there is normal growth of baby and there is no bar for normal delivery. The indications for which caesarean operation is done if also remains in the diabetic pregnant lady, then it is to be done. The decision of mode of delivery is better to leave on obstetrician who is taking care.

69. **Quest**: Whether Insulin is necessary even after delivery?

    Ans: Those who are developed diabetes during pregnancy, on other words, in case of gestational diabetes Insulin is to be stopped. Those who are having diabetes before pregnancy insulin to be continued just like the dose before pregnancy.

70. **Quest**: Whether the diabetic mother can feed breast milk to their baby?

    Ans: Yes, they will feed their baby as other baby gets. But high blood sugar of mother to be controlled by insulin, as insulin is destroyed by acid of stomach of the baby. But the oral anti diabetic medicine those who have insulin secreting affect from pancreas they will also get entry in to the stomach through breast milk and reduce the blood sugar of baby. Hence, it is better to treat mother with insulin till the baby takes breast milk.

71. **Quest**: Please tell something more so that the diabetic lady can successfully become the mother of healthy baby.

    Ans: Most of the points regarding pregnancy and diabetes is discussed above. The highlighted points are as follows:

    a. The diabetic women must plan for pregnancy.

    b. Blood sugar to be controlled by insulin prior to pregnancy.

    c. Before and after pregnancy the diabetic lady should be kept under supervision of a doctor experienced in diabetes.

    d. Regular check up by an experienced obstetrician is also necessary.

    e. To follow the diet plan and exercise as advised is very necessary.

    f. For better control of blood sugar use of self-blood glucose monitor should be used as per advices of doctor.

    If we follow the above-mentioned points, then usually there should not be any obstacle for successful pregnancy.

72. **Quest**: Whether a lady having gestational diabetes may become permanent diabetes or type 2 diabetes in future.

    Ans: Yes, certainly it may appear. Hence, after 6 to 12 weeks of delivery oral glucose tolerance test is advised. And the test to be repeated every 6 months. It is found that in about 30 to 50 percent of cases develops either high value or diabetes.

73. **Quest**: A lady with Type 1 diabetes or childhood diabetes, any special precaution is necessary for pregnancy?

    Ans: They are also to plan for pregnancy. They are to keep blood sugar under control and apart from this, they are to go for special check-up for eyes, kidney, heart to rule out any complication of the vital organs as because the complication becomes more as pregnancy progress and this hamper both mother and baby.

74. **Quest**: Is there any chance of developing diabetes in the baby if blood sugar of mother remains very high?

    Ans: No, such evidence is not there. But because of familial influence of diabetes, it may develop in future at older age.

75. **Quest**: If the male person has high diabetes whether there is any weakness in fertility or chances to produce mal-formed baby?

Ans: No such evidence is there. But it is better to control blood sugar in male person also. If there is weakness in fertility then control of blood sugar may remove the problem. But there is no such evidence of mal-formation of baby.

Diabetes and Monitoring

76. **Quest**: To know about diabetes, which blood sample is preferable?

    Ans: The best is fasting blood sample – 10 to 12 hrs after the last dinner. The normal range is 70 to 100 mg/dl, in diabetes 126 mg/dl and above. In between 101 to 125 mg/dl is impaired fasting glucose or IFB.

77. **Quest**: Sometime it is seen that glucose solution is given before test!

    Ans: Yes, to know blood sugar status definitely – oral glucose tolerance test is done. In this case, after taking blood sample in fasting state as mentioned above, 75 gm of glucose with a glass of water is given (in case of children 1.75 gm/kg of body weight) and in every half an hour interval 4 times blood sample is taken. It is the definitive test for diabetes.

78. **Quest**: What is Random blood sugar?

    Ans: It is the anytime blood sugar. It is necessary if there is symptoms of low blood sugar or in emergency. Apart from this it is usually done in diabetes detection camp. Otherwise, for treatment purpose and dose adjustment it has no such value.

79. **Quest**: Whether one can perform blood sugar test at home?

   Ans: Yes, we can test for sugar at home. We can understand the status of blood sugar by testing urine and blood. There is a good relation with blood sugar and urine sugar. If blood sugar goes above the level of 180 mg/dl then sugar comes out through urine.

80. **Quest**: Then we can test urine sugar without doing blood sugar!

    Ans: If we test blood sugar, we can know the exact level of blood sugar at that time. It is the right way. It is a bit costlier than urine sugar test. Urine is collected in the bladder; hence, urine is to be voided before the time of testing and after few minutes, with second voided urine, sugar test is done and that result has relation with the blood sugar level of that time. If the urine test result is 'nil' then we can say that blood sugar level is below 180 mg/dl, but to know the exact level of blood sugar, blood test is necessary. If the urine sugar test result is trace, 1+,2+ and so on then blood sugar will be high accordingly. At that time, we can omit blood sugar test. Now a days mostly self-blood glucose monitoring is in practice.

81. **Quest**: How urine sugar test is done?

   Ans: We can do urine sugar by two methods-

   1. By Benedict's reagent
   2. By kit method. Benedict's reagent test now is almost obsolete. Kit method is available. It is a readymade strip having reagent in one end. Strip end is rinsed with urine and allowed to rinse for ½ to one minute as mentioned in the container and if urine sugar is present it changes its colour and the colour which matches with the colour mentioned in the container indicating the level of urine sugar as labelled as nil, trace, 1+.2+,3+,4+.

82. **Quest**: Can we measure our blood sugar at home and how?

   Ans: Yes, we can measure our blood sugar by some small digital machine, these are called as Self blood glucose monitor, in short SBGM. We can measure our blood sugar at any time. It is very much essential in hypoglycaemic situation and in situation where control of blood sugar is urgent. Every diabetic person should use this monitor.

83. **Quest**: It is seen that there is a good difference with the value of digital monitor and Laboratory report. Why so?

   Ans: The blood sample collected for SBGM is from tip of the finger and that is capillary blood where as in the laboratory, the blood sample is collected from vein. The glucose content in venous blood and capillary blood differs. The capillary blood is a mixture of both venule and arteriole and contains more sugar than venous blood, the difference becomes more if venous blood sugar becomes more. The Laboratory method is standard. When we go to doctor for check-up, blood sugar to be tested from Laboratory. But at home by doing blood sugar in SBGM machine, we can understand the status of blood sugar about low, normal or high and the results to be noted at note book putting date and time and during check-up it is to be shown to doctor which helps to understand about the status of blood sugar and may help for dose adjustment.

84. **Quest**: If you kindly say something about pre preparation before doing fasting and postprandial (PP) blood sugar.

    Ans Before giving the fasting blood sample, medicine or insulin should not be taken before giving blood. But the day before night, all the medicine should be taken if it is advised. Only water and liquor tea can be taken before giving fasting sample. But for post prandial sample all the medicine before and after meal should be taken as routine. Quantity of meal should be as in daily routine. The time should be counted when the meal is started and at 2 hours blood sample should be given. PP sample may be given after breakfast and after lunch. But the gap between breakfast and lunch should be at least 3 to 4 hours. Water can be taken in between meal and giving blood sample.

85. **Quest**: What is Hba1c test? Is it also a blood sugar test?

    Ans: Hba1c or glycosylated haemoglobin is a product formed after the addition of blood sugar with haemoglobin of RBC of blood. When blood sugar remains high for a longer period of time, there is high level of Hba1c. As the life span of RBC is 120 days, its value gives approximation of previous 3 to 4 months control of blood sugar. Hence, the test is done initially in 3 months interval, later on, when blood sugar becomes control, the test is advised in every 6 months interval.

86. **Quest**: What other tests are necessary along with test for blood sugar?

    Ans: The following tests are necessary along with blood sugar test:

    a. Routine test for urine: A lot of information we can gather from this test. Urinary albumin has a direct relation with status of kidney disease.

    b. Micro albumin test of Urine: If albumin is absent in routine test of urine then Micro albumin test is necessary. Micro albumin is the early marker of kidney disease.

c. Urine test after 24 hrs. collection of urine – It is done after 24 hours collection of urine.

d. Routine blood examination: It is done as other diseases. A lot of information is gathered about health status and disease.

e. Blood Creatinine level: Serum Creatinine level is very urgent to understand the status of kidney disease. Its normal value usually 0.6 to 1.2 mg/dl. In kidney failure it becomes 4 mg/dl or above. In between 1.2 and 4 mg/dl – it is the state of renal insufficiency.

f. Blood Lipid profile: We can gather status of blood fat as cholesterol and other fats. If it is found to be normal then test to be repeated after 6 months.

g. Chest X-ray: As the incidence of lungs TB is more in diabetes, it is to be done in 1st visit.

h. ECG: With this test we can understand about the heart disease. So, it is to be done in initial one or two visits.

i. Eye test: Complete eye test should be done in initial visits specially in Type 2 diabetes. If there is any defect, check-up should be done as per direction of doctor. If it is normal check-up should be done every year.

j. Apart from these tests, doctor will advise necessary test if and when required.

Diabetes and Hypoglycaemia

87. **Quest**: What is hypoglycaemia?

    Ans: When blood sugar comes down below 70 mg/dl, it is said to be hypoglycaemia. But when the blood sugar comes down below 55 mg/dl, symptoms of hypoglycaemia express as excess hunger, excess sweating, palpitation, feeling of tremor, haziness, giddiness, headache and many uneasiness symptoms. These symptoms become more as time passes and gradually becomes stupor to unconsciousness. This stage is called Hypoglycaemic coma. The treatment should be done urgently and immediately.

88. **Quest**: Why hypoglycaemia occurs?

    Ans: Hypoglycaemia occurs in diabetes for the following reasons:

    a. If the dose of medicine becomes more.

    b. When one remains fasting for longer time or takes little amount of food then the required amount.

c. When patient works hard for longer time.

   d. If there is vomiting or diarrhoea.

89. **Quest**: If it is so, then the treatment of diabetes is a tough job. It may happen in every patient at any time. And it is not always possible to bring the patient to a doctor!

    Ans: Yes, it may happen in every diabetic patient at any time. Whenever there is feeling of excess hunger, palpitation, tremor etc then it is to be assumed that blood sugar is getting down and food should be taken immediately available nearby. Thus, the symptom subsides by this simple mean. Some time, though the symptoms subsides but the weakness last for few hours.

90. **Quest**: Whether Hypoglycaemia happens again and again?

    Ans: Yes, it may repeat. Hence it is to be inquired why it happens? If the cause is due to food, then food should be taken in right time and in right quantity. If food is OK, then the dose of medicine should be reduced and letter on the dose should be adjusted by consulting doctor. If there is vomiting or diarrhoea, immediate consultation with doctor is necessary.

91. **Quest**: When a patient goes to a stage of unconsciousness due to low sugar, then it is

very difficult to feed sugar-water. What is to be done at that time?

Ans: In such situation, the patient should be transferred immediately to a hospital, nursing home or to a doctor without any delay and information about diabetes and medicine should be told. Then Doctor can straightway think of low blood sugar and start treatment without wasting time to inquire and investigate the other probable causes of unconsciousness. Usually, 100 cc of 25% glucose through IV route is given quickly. Patients regains consciousness on treatment but sooner the better.

92. **Quest**: Is it very urgent to test for blood sugar during low sugar?

    Ans: If test can be done as urgent, it should be done. Otherwise, it is better to push IV 25% glucose without wasting time. If it is due to low blood sugar, it will save the patient. If it is other than low blood sugar, this glucose injection will not harm the patient.

93. **Quest**: You have advised to reduce dose of medicine if there is low blood sugar when the food is OK. Is it necessary to check blood sugar before reducing the dose?

    Ans: When there is symptom of low blood sugar, if glucometer is available it is better to check blood sugar. If the glucometer is not available, then it is better to take food immediately available nearby without going to a doctor or laboratory. Some time it is seen that after low sugar symptoms if blood sugar test is done the figure becomes extra ordinary high. It is because when there is low blood sugar body releases excess amount of sugar from the stored food (glycogen) in the body. This phenomenon is called Somogyi effect. Hence, after low sugar symptoms, one should not be puzzled after observing high blood sugar. Hence, measured should be taken as per symptom of low sugar.

94. **Quest**: Whether it may so happen that when there is hypoglycaemia and the person cannot recognise? If it is so, why it happens and how to overcome the problem?

    Ans: It may happen. It usually happens when there is abnormality in autonomic nervous system (autonomic neuropathy) which usually regulates internal environment. In established autonomic neuropathy there is failure of normal reaction caused by hypoglycaemia and lead to brain cell damage, fits and seizure, coma and even death. If it develops in sleep, it is very danger. Alcoholism also disturbs the glucose regulation by inhibiting glucagon breakdown to sugar. Autonomic neuropathy usually takes place in long standing uncontrolled diabetes and recurring episodes of hypoglycaemia. To prevent hypoglycaemic problem, only way is to take regular meals and to take snacks in between two major meals in

2–3 hrs. intervals. Frequent checking of blood sugar with SBGM and awareness among family members is very necessary.

95. **Quest**: Will you kindly say something more so that one can avoid danger out of low sugar?

    Ans: First important thing is that every diabetic person should carry a diabetes identity card – which will bear the name of the patient, address, contact no, name of the doctor, contact no, diagnosis and type of medicine one is taking and some sort of directions which should one to follow. If one bears the card, anybody can help in crisis. Other points are:

    a. Regular intake of medicine in time

    b. Never skip meal.

    c. To consult with doctor in any sort of illness.

    d. Regular check-up as advised by doctor.

    e. Let everybody specially people of working place to know about his/her diabetes and about low sugar symptoms and what to do in low blood sugar and hypoglycaemic coma.

    f. Dose of diabetic medicine should not be increased in any circumstances without consulting doctor.

    g. Everybody should carry some dry type of foods having high carbohydrate as sugar-candy, chocolate, biscuits and water, so that one can take if feels hungry.

h. Thus, if the person or the guardian of a diabetic child becomes a bit alert, then the crisis of low sugar can easily be avoided.

96. **Quest**: In high blood sugar also patient feels uneasiness, even becomes unconscious!

Ans: Yes, it is true. It happens in two special conditions: 1) Diabetic ketoacidosis and 2) Hyperosmolar diabetes nonketotic coma. Diabetes keto acidosis usually occurs, in case of children having Type 1 diabetes if remains undetected or stops insulin and usually associates with other diseases. In such case, ketone level in blood increases along with blood sugar. In the urine there is high amount of acetone and in the breath out air, there is smell of fruits. The second situation happens usually in the older one. Most of the time, this happens due to negligence. Blood sugar becomes extremely high, even becomes above 600mg/dl, leading to dry mouth, raised body temperature, feeling drowsiness and even senseless. Both the conditions are to be dealt with emergency.

Diabetes and Complication

97. **Quest**: Sometime it is seen that in diabetic patient, the wound heals in normal duration but sometime delayed. Why it is so?

    Ans: If the blood sugar remains in control, the wound heals normally. When blood sugar remains high for long time, specially, if fasting blood sugar remains around 200 mg/dl or more then due to glycation of protein, the function of blood cells become impaired. The oxygen carrying capacity of RBC and fighting action of WBC becomes impaired and causes delayed wound healing.

98. **Quest**: Diabetic people occasionally gets haziness of vision and power of lens of spectacles needs to be changed. Why it is so?

    Ans: In every eye there is a lens and it is a biological lens. When blood sugar remains high, the water from lens comes out and lens contracted and the light cannot reach the retina, the biological screen; again, when the blood sugar becomes low, the water enters into the lens and lens becomes expanded and the light focuses beyond retina. Hence, when there is high blood sugar or low blood sugar or blood sugar is unstable, the vision becomes blurred. That is why, the power of lens of spectacle should not be changed till the blood sugar becomes normal and stable.

99. **Quest**: Sometime peoples complains of black spot or light particle moving around?

    Ans: Yes, it may happen when there is minute bleeding from abnormal vessels of retina (Retinopathy) which floats in the fluids of eye ball. If there is excess bleeding there may be sudden loss of vision.

100. **Quest**: Is it inevitable for every diabetic patient? Can it be prevented?

    Ans: If blood sugar remains uncontrolled, then in Type 1 diabetes, retinopathy develop after 5 to 10 years of detection but in Type 2 diabetes it may appear very early even at the time of first detection. There is no relation with the power of lens or haziness of vision. So, every diabetic person should undergo eye check-up for retinopathy. This retinopathy becomes more denser with times. If there is high blood pressure along with uncontrolled diabetes then the retina becomes more vulnerable. Thus, for prevention we should be careful about:

a. Eye test should be done at the time of detection of type 2 diabetes. But in type 1 diabetes it should be done after 5 yrs of detection. If remains normal, then it should be done in every 6 months.

b. keeping blood sugar under control.

c. keeping high blood pressure under control.

d. To avoid tobacco of any form.

e. If there is retinopathy, it should be treated with Eye specialist having experienced with retinopathy.

101. **Quest:** What is laser treatment? Is it operation? With this Laser treatment does the retina becomes alright?

    Ans: There are so many stages of retinopathy. When it advances then few tiny vessels of retina become flattens (aneurysm) and there is formation of very thin-walled new vessels which bleeds. These vessels are blocked by laser treatment preventing bleeding. But similar situation may develop if blood sugar and blood pressure remain uncontrolled. Thus, it requires 3 to 6 monthly check up or as advised by doctor. Laser treatment is done through a special device, it does not require any incision or hospitalization.

102. **Quest**: Is there any relation with diabetic kidney disease and retinopathy?

    Ans: Yes, the abnormality of small blood vessels develops in every organ as in retinopathy. It is observed that the chronic kidney disease develops in about 35% of cases. The diabetic kidney disease is first detected when there is leakage of protein. Then gradually intensify. If precaution is taken from the early phage, the disease can be prevented or postponed.

103. **Quest**: Sometime amputation of leg is done in diabetic people.

    Ans: In diabetic people, there is disease of both small and big vessels and in foot, there is influence of both type of vessels disease. Again, there is impaired sensations due peripheral nerve disease. We also take least care for the feet. So, if there is injury on foot, immediate care should be taken. If it is seen that there is impaired blood circulation and wound is not healing through proper treatment, rather infection progresses and then decision of amputation should be taken without hesitation to save the limb as far as possible.

104. **Quest**: What are the preventive measures we can take to avoid diabetic complication?

    Ans: Uncontrolled blood sugar produces diabetic complications. The other factors which enhance complications are high blood pressure, high blood cholesterol, obesity, tobacco use, and idle life style. So, to prevent diabetic complication the measures are:

a. To control of blood sugar – Fasting blood sugar from 80 mg/dl to 120 mg/dl, Postprandial blood sugar (2 hr after meal) from 120 mg/dl to 160 mg/dl and Glycated haemoglobin below 7%.

b. blood cholesterol level should be kept below 200 mg/dl.

c. Blood pressure level below 130/80 mm of Hg.

d. Body weight should be kept around ideal body wt.

e. To avoid any form of tobacco.

f. To lead an active life with proper exercise.

g. If we can maintain all the above things then it is possible to prevent and postpone the diabetic complication.

105. **Quest**: When there is complication due to diabetes, is it necessary to treat the patient with insulin.

Ans: It is not mandatory. So many agents are available now a days. But Insulin is the best. Main target is to keep blood sugar under control. If there is other diseases of vital organ as Liver disease (Jaundice), Nephritis etc blood sugar should be controlled with Insulin as a temporary measure.

106. **Quest**: Bad influence of diabetes on eyes and kidney is developing slowly. Is it possible reversed back to normal from any stage? Is it possible at all?

    Ans: Bad influence on kidney in type 1 diabetes starts after 5 years from detection. Of course, if there is high blood pressure also then it may happen early. In type 2 diabetes it may be seen even at the time of detection of diabetes. Hence, in case of type 2 diabetes, test for kidney and eyes should be performed in the initial visits. If there is no abnormality, then albumin test in urine should be performed in every visit if possible. Micro albumin is the early marker of kidney disease. If it progresses, albumin will be detected. Then creatinine level of blood increases. Normal level of creatinine level is below 1.4 mg/dl. When it crosses 4 mg/dl, then it is the stage of renal failure. The stage between 1.4 mg/dl to 4 mg/dl is called as Renal insufficiency. When there is presence of micro albumin, intensification of care should be taken. When there is albumin level in the urine around 500 mg/24 hr, from that stage with proper treatment it is possible to bring back to normal. When there is detection of micro albumin in urine, test for eyes and heart should be performed. If there is renal failure, the dialysis should be performed and preparation for kidney transplant should be initiated.

107. **Quest**: Many a time it is observed that the diabetic people suffer from sexual disability disturbing conjugal life. Is it for diabetes?

    Ans: Yes, it may happen. In long term uncontrolled diabetes, there is weakness in nerves. Again, there may be deposition of fat inside the blood vessels of sex organs (Atherosclerosis) disturbing blood flow and sexual inabilities. If treatment is done in initial phage, it can be rectified. Most of the time it happens due to physical weakness and mentally stressed condition and can be return back to normal with treatment and counselling.

108. **Quest**: Whether sexual disability happens in both male and female?

    Ans: Yes, it may develop in both cases. But, in sexual activity, most of the time, as males are taking active role, so male's inability are becoming pronounced.

109. **Quest**: Whether the diabetic will restrict their sexual activities?

    Ans: No, it should be normal as desire. It is better to keep relation with proper understanding between the couples. For sexual activity it is better to hand over on female partner. When female partner desires, then both are getting real satisfaction. If any abnormality is observed in any of the partner, it is better to discuss between and consult with doctor.

110. **Quest**: Sometime it is found that there is foul smell from mouth, dental pain and bleeding from gum in many of diabetics!

    Ans: Yes, it may happen. When there is high blood sugar, then the saliva also contains high sugar which facilitates growth of bacteria and thus produces foul smell, dental disease and gum disease. Thus, along with control of blood sugar, oral hygiene is also to be maintained by regular brushing specially after dinner. If necessary, consultation with dentist should be done.

111. **Quest**: Many a time, it is found that a number of diabetic people do suffer from Chest TB!

    Ans: Yes, the diabetics are more prone to get Tuberculosis of Lungs. The main causes are:

    1. Poor nutrition,

    2. Poor oxygen carrying capacity of blood cells,

    3. Poor resistance power of the body,

    4. High sugar facilitates bacterial growth. The diabetics also develop nerve weakness for which the primary symptoms of disease remain unnoticed. Hence, in the initial visits – the chest X-ray and other investigations is done for ruling out tuberculosis.

112. **Quest**: Heart disease is also more with Diabetes!

    Ans: The heart disease is more with diabetic then with non-diabetic and the rate increases by 2 to 3 folds. If there is high blood pressure, high cholesterol or use of any form of tobacco is there along with diabetes then the rate of cardiac disease and stroke increases with many folds. So along with control of diabetes high blood pressure, high cholesterol and using of tobacco also to be controlled.

113. **Quest**: Is it inevitable that any sort of complication will develop in diabetics?

    Ans: No, it cannot be said specially in Type 2 diabetes. If everything is under control, then scope of developing complication is reduced very much. But in Type 1 diabetes, it is very difficult to control diabetes in the running method of treatment and it is very difficult to prevent complication.

114. **Quest**: Commonly it is seen that the people with Type 2 diabetes suffer from stroke and coronary heart disease and those who are of type 1 diabetes suffer from Kidney failure. Why it is so?

    Ans: As mentioned earlier, blood vessels disease is of two types – small vessel disease (Micro vascular) and large vessels disease

(Macro vascular). Diabetic kidney disease is due to small vessels disease and Heart disease as heart attack and stroke (in brain) is due to large vessels disease. Small vessels disease depends on high blood sugar where as large vessels disease depends on high blood sugar, high cholesterol, high pressure and so on. As Type 1 diabetes usually occurs in childhood age and control of blood sugar is very difficult, hence, kidney disease starts after 5 to 10 years of starting diabetes, and progresses gradually towards end stage. Where as in Type 2 diabetes, the patient preserves some insulin secreting cells and with treatment blood sugar can be controlled. The large vessels disease starts some time even before the diagnosis of Type 2 diabetes and with the influence of lipid and other factors large vessels disease advances and develop heart attack, stroke etc.

115. **Quest**: Why foot care is important in diabetes?

Ans: The foot is vulnerable to get injury and infected with dirt. Again, due to blood vessels disease, blood supply in the limbs may be impaired and due to weakness of nerve (neuropathy) there is impaired sensation. Patient ignores mild injury for impaired sensation. And antibacterial agent cannot reach at the infected site due to blockage on vessels, thus, infection spreads rapidly and forms gangrene and septic condition of the leg.

116. **Quest**: What are the points to be observed in foot care?

    Ans: The following main points to be observed in caring foot:

    a. While walking on road, one should wear shoes and socks. Shoes should not be too loose nor too tight, it must be well fitted and comfort. New shoes should be broken gradually to avoid frictional injury or blister.

    b. If there is injury on foot, urgent care should be taken and doctor should be consulted if necessary.

    c. During cutting nail, one should soften the nail after rinsing or nail should be cut after taking bath. Nail cutter should be used instead of shaving blade.

    d. The feet should be cleaned every night thoroughly and after drying with clean towel or cotton cloth, any talcum powder should be applied on foot specially in between toes in summer where as in winter some body lotion, oil or moisturizing cream should be applied to avoid crack.

    e. Foot should be observed daily at night for any injury, impaired sensation or change in colour of the skin. If any abnormality is observed, doctor should be consulted.

f. Sometime, callus appears on sole and consultation with doctor is required. These are the few important points. It is said that in diabetes, foot care is more impotent then care of face.

Diabetes and Obesity

117. **Quest**: Most of the time it is seen that the obese people become diabetic. What is the relation?

    Ans: Over Weight or obesity, most of the time, as if the preliminary stage of diabetes. Usually, family history of diabetes is present. All the obese person will develop diabetes is not true.

118. **Quest**: Are all the fat man obese? Who are actually obese?

    Ans: The stage of body weight is determined by body mass index, in short BMI. The formula of determining BMI = weight in kg / (height in meter)2(square). For example. If body weight is 60 kg and height is 1.6 meter. Then BMI is 60/1.6*1.6= 23.4. A man will be underweight if his BMI is less than 18.5, Normal weight BMI is 18.5 to 24.9, Over weight if BMI is 25 to 29.9 and obese if BMI is 30 and above.

119. **Quest**: What other problems one may face with obesity?

Ans: The highly obese person normally face difficulty in movement. High blood pressure and diabetes is more among obese person. Apart from these, heart attack, stroke, decreased libido is more due to atherosclerosis in obese people. Fracture of bone, mental depression, impaired memory, even cancer is more in obese people. Hence, body weight should be maintained nearest to ideal body weight.

120. **Quest**: It is more often seen that all the people of a family are obese. Is it due to hereditary influence?

Ans: It cannot be truly said that it is due to hereditary influence. Mostly, it is due to similar lifestyle as dietary habit, physical inactivity etc. of the family.

Diabetes and Special Situations

121. **Quest**: During sick days specially in fever, gastro enteritis etc. when the person cannot take food normally, do they continue anti diabetic medicine as before or reduced the dose.

    Ans: During disease, there is stress in the body. During stress there is increase in insulin resistance and demands more insulin. Thus, the dose of antidiabetic medicine should not be reduced. Rather, treatment for the disease is urgently needed. The food or alternate food should be encouraged as in nondiabetic person. If not possible, then patient should be admitted and IV route should be chosen.

122. **Quest**: Many a person used to practice fast mostly in religious purpose as in 'Upobas' and in Ramadan or 'ROSA'. Whether any adjustment of dose require?

    Ans: There are many types of fasting. Sometime without taking anything, even not taking water for a whole day and night, sometime for certain period of time, sometime used to take very small quantity of liquid type of food. The diabetic patient should not go for fast for long time. It may cause harm. In uncontrolled diabetes, it is better to avoid total fast for longer period. During ROSA and fasting for a number of days, the type of medicine and dose of medicine require adjustment.

123. **Quest**: During feast in festival or invitation, whether antidiabetic medicine require higher dose?

    Ans: No, in no way, dose of medicine should be increased. Rather it is better to choose items what usually fits. Some sort of alteration of food with limitation may be done.

124. **Quest**: During travel, whether the change of medicine or dose reduction is required?

    Ans: Not necessary. Where ever we go, we are to eat. The time may differ a bit. Most of the medicine are used to take before or after food. Hence, whenever we are taking meal, we are to take medicine. We should not search for food after taking medicine. Rather, when the meal is ready, we are to take medicine. In special situation, we can take medicine just before meal or after meal. It does not matter much. If there is delay of getting meal, we are to take extra snacks on that time to avoid feeling hunger.

During travel, one should carry – doctor's prescription, sufficient amount of medicine. In case of insulin, insulin should be carried in handbag and no need to keep in fridge.

125. **Quest**: During game and tournament, a participant has to work for longer time. How medicine and diet should be adjusted?

    Ans: No adjustment of dose of medicine is required. The diet should be as usual. Only thing is that as the participant has to work for longer time and burns lot of calorie, the participant has to take high carbohydrate, easy digestible snacks or drinks in between to avoid low sugar as well as to maintain calorie for work.

126. **Quest**: Any comment on alcoholic beverages?

    Ans: When a person is having tight control of blood sugar, alcoholic beverage brings the blood sugar down and natural way to prevent hypoglycaemia is also disturbed, even symptoms of hypoglycaemia remain unexpressed. It is a danger situation. On the other hand, those who are having uncontrolled and high blood sugar, alcoholic drinks cause more difficult to control diabetes. Hence, alcoholic drinks are in no way good for diabetes. But those who are occasional drinker, a little amount of wine with water or non-sugar soda can be taken. Those who are habituated, a limited quantity of 1 to 2 pegs is allowed. High alcoholic drink also causes high triglyceride level and peripheral neuropathy, alcoholic hepatitis etc.

Diabetes and Future

127. **Quest**: What is the future of Diabetes?

    Ans: We know that 90% of total diabetics are of Type 2 diabetes and strong hereditary influence is responsible for this. Hence, number of Type 2 diabetes will increase with days. On the other hand, in Type 1 diabetes, though we cannot deny the hereditary influence but other disease or factors are responsible for this. If we can detect this disease and factors properly and can prevent by treatment and vaccine, then there is a chance to reduce the rate of Type 1 diabetes. When the transplantation of beta cells of pancreas can be done successfully without having side effect, then there will be dramatic relief for type 1 diabetes. But for Type 2 diabetes good life style will be the only procedure for prevention. As Type 2 diabetes depends on hereditary influence, so pre matrimonial counselling as other hereditary disease may be necessary. And the number of children of diabetic family to be minimized. A part from this, everyone should perform regular exercise, daily physical labour, understanding and acceptance of scientifically well-balanced diet, sufficient rest and sleep, avoidance of all sorts of tobacco and other addicting substances and maintaining good conjugal life, and good social relation are the back bone of good health preventing diabetes and its complication, heart attack, stroke, cancer, AIDS, depressive disorder and many other diseases.

128. **Quest**: Which organization primarily regulates activities on Diabetes?

Ans: World health organization (WHO) primarily acts as chief regulator. But IDF (International Diabetes federation) specially deals with Diabetes. In India, Diabetes association of India has been working on awareness program on Diabetes in general population since 1955. RSSDI works mainly on Diabetes research in India.

129. **Quest**: What is blue Circle? Is it associated with Diabetes?

Ans: Yes, Diabetes has become endemic all over the world. Its impact on society is also fatal and render burden on family and society as a whole. Hence, every man and woman in this world require heart felt will to control it. Thus, the blue circle is formed with the blue colour of sky indicating vastness. Blue circle is as if declaring – "Global unity to control Diabetes pandemic".

www.ingramcontent.com/pod-product-compliance
Lightning Source LLC
Chambersburg PA
CBHW020930180526
45163CB00007B/2965